Changes
Contents

Solids, liquids and gases	5	Making compost	20
Changing solids, liquids and gases	6	Genetics	21
Separating substances	7	Fossils	22
Dissolving things	8	Changes in the landscape – 1	23
Physical and chemical changes	9	Weathering	24
Making chemical changes	10	Changes in the landscape – 2	25
Manufactured changes	11	The water cycle	26
Changing colours	12	Changes in the weather – temperature	27
Chromatography	13	Changes in the weather – wind speed and rainfall	28
Changing sounds	14		
Changes in strength	15	Changes in the weather – wind direction	29
Animal life cycles	16	The seasons	30
How plants change	17	Day and night	31
Photosynthesis	18	Changes in the moon	32
Will it rot?	19		

Teachers' notes

The aims of this book
▲ To introduce the notion of change in the world around us.
▲ To promote awareness of physical and chemical changes, both in the natural world and in human activities.
▲ To provide experience in observing, predicting, recording, measuring and making hypotheses.
▲ To provide opportunities for children to share their ideas with others.

Developing science skills
While it is not necessary to follow the order of the worksheets, it is important that all those covering one aspect of the subject, such as the weather, are dealt with at approximately the same time.

Although it is in the doing of science that children learn best, this involves more than just practical work. They need to observe, record, predict, measure, look for patterns, classify, explain and ask questions that can lead to further investigations. They need time to discuss their work, before and after the activity; this will also aid the teacher in monitoring the children's progress so that they build a valid framework for future development.

Safety precautions
All the activities described in this book use everyday equipment and materials which are perfectly safe if used sensibly. If extra care is needed on some activities, this is mentioned in the body of the worksheet and again in these notes.

Scientific background
Scientific background information has been provided in the teachers' notes to help you understand the scientific concepts and ideas covered. It generally goes beyond the level of understanding of most children, but will give you the confidence to ask and answer questions and guide the children in their investigations.

Page 5: Solids, liquids and gases
Key idea: To introduce the terms *solid, liquid* and *gas*.
Scientific background: The molecules in solids stay in one position, hence solids can maintain a definite shape. The molecules in a liquid stay close together, but move about. The molecules in a gas move about very rapidly and rebound from one another.
Likely outcome: butter – solid; honey – liquid; wood – solid; bubbles – gas; inside a balloon – gas; salt – solid; ice lolly – solid; candle – solid; ketchup – liquid; paper – solid; steam – gas; nail – solid.

Page 6: Changing solids, liquids and gases
Key idea: To investigate the changes of matter.
Scientific background: Applying heat causes molecules to move faster, hence a solid can be turned into a liquid and liquid into a gas. Vinegar (an acid) will react with baking powder to form carbon dioxide.
Likely outcome: Water boiled turns to steam (gas), fruit juice frozen turns to ice (solid), baking powder and vinegar form carbon dioxide (gas), butter heated melts (liquid), sugar dissolves in hot water (liquid).
Safety precaution: Ensure the kettle lead is out of reach. Do not let children use boiling water unsupervised.

▲ ESSENTIALS FOR SCIENCE: Changes

Extension: Investigate other changes of state – do all solids melt? Can all liquids freeze? and so on.

Page 7: Separating substances

Key idea: How filters can clean water.
Scientific background: Filtration involves the use of a barrier to hold back particles of solids. Groundwater is filtered as it passes through layers of rocks and soil. The solution passing through the filter is called the filtrate, insoluble material on the filter is the residue.
Likely outcome: The muddy water will become clear as it filters through. Finer filters are more effective.
Extension: Filter a variety of waters, e.g. tap, pond, river, mineral, to find out which is the cleanest.

Page 8: Dissolving things

Key idea: Dissolving substances in water.
Scientific background: Not all substances dissolve in water and some only partially dissolve. Heating increases the rate of dissolving. Fine powders dissolve more quickly than coarse ones. Water is called the solvent and the substance dissolved is called the solute. Solvent + solute = solution.
Likely outcome: Sugar and salt will dissolve; pepper flour and scouring powder will not dissolve; bicarbonate of soda will partially dissolve.
Extension: Investigate other solvents, e.g. turpentine will dissolve fats and oils that will not dissolve in water.

Page 9: Physical and chemical changes

Key idea: To differentiate between physical and chemical changes.
Scientific background: In a physical change no new substance is formed or destroyed, there is no change in weight, it can usually be reversed easily and the energy changes are usually small. In chemical changes, the substance is changed and new substances are formed, there is a change in weight, a reverse change is difficult and the energy changes are often large.
Likely outcome: The ice lolly, wood, drink can and heated milk undergo a physical change, while the yoghurt and bread are the result of chemical changes.

Page 10: Making chemical changes

Key idea: Chemical changes in substances.
Scientific background: Steel is mostly iron. Iron combines with oxygen in the air to form iron oxide (rust). Water helps to speed up the chemical action. As wood burns, water, carbon dioxide, methane, pentane, hexane and octane are produced.
Likely outcome: The steel wool will rust, the matchstick turns to charcoal and the paper to ash.

Page 11: Manufactured changes

Key idea: To differentiate between a raw material and a manufactured material.
Likely outcome: Raw materials – diamond, oil, iron ore, gold, wool, coal, salt, milk and silk. Glass, steel, plastic, flour, aluminium and petrol are manufactured.
Extension: Make a list of raw and manufactured materials in the classroom. Find out where the raw materials come from in the world and how they are made into manufactured products.

Page 12: Changing colours

Key ideas: Mixing primary colours and mixing shades of colour. To mix colours through spinning.
Scientific background: Different (secondary) colours can be made using the three primary colours – red, yellow and blue. White light is made up of all the colours of the rainbow. We see an object as being a certain colour because that colour is reflected by the object. In a spinning disc, your eyes are deceived because they cannot pick out the separate colours. If the disc was painted the seven colours of the rainbow, it would look white when spun.
Likely outcome: blue and yellow – green; red and yellow – orange; red and blue – purple; red, blue and yellow – dirty brown; blue and white – light blue; red and white – pink; yellow and white – light yellow, cream.

Page 13: Chromatography

Key idea: How one colour is made up of different colours.
Scientific background: Some colours will quickly spread out, others will move slowly.
Extension: Try different water temperatures.

Page 14: Changing sounds

Key idea: Changing musical sounds.
Scientific background: Sound is caused by vibrations. Blowing across the top of a bottle causes the air inside the bottle to vibrate. Differences in pitch are caused by the amount of water inside and the type of bottle used (less mass of air = higher pitch).
Likely outcome: Different amounts of water, different lengths and thicknesses of rubber bands and differing amounts and types of beads inside a container will produce different sounds.
Extension: Make a class band with hitting, shaking, plucking, beating and blowing instruments.

Page 15: Changes in strength

Key idea: How to make paper stronger.
Likely outcome: Paper which is folded or rolled will be much stronger than flat paper.
Extension: Make a bridge from newspaper which will stand and has the longest span.

Page 16: Animal life cycles

Key idea: To observe the stages in life cycles.
Extension: Find out about more difficult insects such as butterflies.
Note: Check with the LEA about keeping animals in classrooms; some do not allow tadpoles to be taken from ponds. Mealworms are excellent for observing all stages of the life cycle at once. They can be obtained from pet shops and are easy to maintain.

Page 17: How plants change

Key idea: The various stages of growth of a bean plant.
Likely outcome: Bean seed, seed with small root, seed with long root and small shoot, longer roots and shoot, tall plant, tall plant with flowers, tall plant with some flowers dead and a few small bean pods, tall plant with most flowers dead and more bean pods, tall plant with large bean pods.
Extension: Grow bean seeds under different conditions such as in shade, in the dark, with water, without water, in soil, in sand.

Page 18: Photosynthesis

Key idea: How photosynthesis works.
Likely outcome: The covered leaves will be lighter in colour than the other leaves. The amount of photosynthesis depends on the amount of light energy received. When testing for starch, the part of the leaf exposed to light becomes coloured by the iodine due to the presence of starch. Bubbles of oxygen are produced by the pondweed when in sunlight, less bubbles are produced when in the dark.

Page 19: Will it rot?

Key idea: To investigate food decay, mould growth.
Safety precautions: Do not open the bags once they are prepared as spores from mould are harmful.
Likely outcome: Food which is damp, warm or dirty (wiped on the floor) will go mouldy more quickly.
Extension: Discuss safe food handling and hygiene.

Page 20: Making compost

Key idea: To have firsthand experience of making compost; to investigate the use of compost.
Scientific background: Decay occurs due to decomposers such as bacteria, fungi and earthworms. The processes involved produce heat and the compost can steam. The smell produced by rotting food is caused by the nitrogen- and sulphur-compounds formed.
Likely outcome: The compost becomes dark and crumbly. The seed planted in compost will grow better than the other.
Extension: Find out about other recycling/reusing processes and environmental issues.

Page 21: Genetics

Key idea: Certain characteristics are inherited.
Scientific background: We inherit genes for certain traits from one parent and genes for other traits from the other parent. Some traits are dominant and others are recessive and this determines which parental trait is inherited.
Likely outcome: Eyes – dark/hazel and green are dominant; hair – dark is dominant; freckles are dominant; ear lobes – free is dominant; nose – turned up is dominant. Be aware of children who may not know their real parents.
Extension: Explore evolutionary changes from dinosaurs to modern-day creatures.

Page 22: Fossils

Key idea: To illustrate how fossils are formed.
Extension: Visit places where fossils are found. Make a 'dig' in the school grounds. Find out how fossils tell us how creatures have changed over time.

Page 23: Changes in the landscape – 1

Key idea: How erosion affects the landscape.
Likely outcome: 1 – water erosion: water wears away at the weaker rocks forming cracks and holes. These enlarge into caves, which in turn eventually form an arch. A stack is formed when the roof of the arch collapses. 2 – wind and water: in deserts, water comes from torrential downpours which causes very steep canyons. Plateaux wear away into mesas, then buttes. Sand dunes are caused by the wind. 3 – ice erosion: the gradual, more even wearing away of the glacier forms a rounded valley. Harder rock forms ridges, lakes and waterfalls.
Extension: Find out about river and coastal erosion.

Page 24: Weathering

Key idea: To show how acid rain wears away rocks.
Likely outcome: The surface of the chalk soaked in acid will become pitted and worn. The acid will make this piece of chalk easier to break.
Extension: Discuss acid rain and environmental issues.

Page 25: Changes in the landscape – 2

Key idea: To provide opportunities to discuss the effects humans have on the landscape.
Likely outcome: 1 – positive: jobs created, improved transport network; negative: pollution from factories and cars, wildlife habitats destroyed, farm land decreased. 2 – positive: wildlife habitats created, pollution cleaned up, recreation place created. 3 – positive: more homes provided, jobs created; negative: farming land destroyed, wildlife habitats destroyed, pollution from household wastes, cars and so on.
Extension: Discuss the environmental impact of humans – ozone layer, greenhouse effect, pollution.

Page 26: The water cycle

Key idea: To introduce the concept of the water cycle and how water is used by humans.
Likely outcome: 1 – evaporation, 2 – water vapour, 3 – condensation, 4 – precipitation, 5 – runoff, 6 – groundwater, 7 – irrigation, 8 – purification, 9 – evaporation.
Extension: Demonstrate how rain is made by boiling a kettle and holding a tray of ice above the steam. Water will condense and drops of 'rain' will fall.

Page 27: Changes in the weather – temperature

Key idea: To investigate changes in air temperature.
Likely outcome: The air temperature will be cooler in the shade and warmer at the middle of the day.
Extension: Investigate the 'chill factor', placing some thermometers in the wind and some out of the wind.

Page 28: Changes in the weather – wind speed and rainfall

Key idea: To measure wind speed and rainfall.
Scientific background: Wind is moving air. It moves from high to low pressure areas. The greater the difference between the high and low pressure, the greater the quantity and speed of air moved. Rain is formed by water which evaporates from lakes and oceans. This condenses and forms clouds when the water vapour cools, droplets then fall as rain.

Page 29: Changes in the weather – wind direction

Key idea: To investigate how wind changes direction.
Likely outcome: The wind vane should demonstrate a prevailing wind direction for your area.

Page 30: The seasons

Key idea: How the seasons affect plants and animals.
Likely outcome: Autumn: hedgehog – hibernates, beech – loses leaves. Winter: holly – produces berries, stoat – coat changes to white. Spring: swallow – returns to Britain from Africa, daffodil – flowers. Summer: grass – grows quickly, salmon – migrate upstream to spawn.
Extension: Look at other plants and animals.

Page 31: Day and night

Key idea: The changes which occur to the environment during the day and night.
Likely outcome: The hours of daylight will depend on the season – more in summer than in winter.
Extension: Demonstrate how night and day are created using a lamp and a globe.

Page 32: Changes in the moon

Key idea: Why the moon changes shape.
Likely outcome:

crescent	
first quarter (half)	gibbous
full	gibbous
last quarter (half)	crescent

National Curriculum: Science

In addition to the PoS for AT1, the following PoS are relevant to this book:
AT2 – Pupils should:
• investigate the factors that affect plant growth, for example light intensity, temperature and amount of water;
• find out how animals and plants are influenced by environmental conditions including seasonal and daily changes;
• study aspects of the local environment affected by human activity, for example, farming, industry, mining or quarrying and consider the benefits and detrimental effects of these activities;
• investigate the key factors in the process of decay, such as temperature, moisture, air and the role of microbes;
AT3 – Pupils should:
• compare a range of solids, liquids and gases and recognise the properties which enable classification of materials in this way;
• develop ideas about solutions and solubility through experiments on dissolving and evaporation;
• explore ways to separate and purify mixtures such as muddy or salty water and ink, by evaporation, filtration and chromatography;
• explore the origins of materials in order to appreciate that some occur naturally while many are made from raw materials.
• investigate the action of heat on everyday materials resulting in permanent change;
• explore chemical changes in a number of everyday materials such as those which occur when mixing plaster of Paris, mixing baking powder with vinegar and when iron rusts;
• observe, through fieldwork, how weather affects their surroundings.
AT4 – Pupils should:
• investigate changes that occur when familiar substances are heated and cooled;
• investigate the strength of a simple structure;
• learn that sounds are made when objects vibrate, and investigate how sounds are changed in pitch, loudness and timbre;
• learn about the motions of the Earth, Moon and Sun in order to explain day and night, phases of the moon and the seasons.

Scottish Curriculum 5–14: Science

Attainment outcome	Strand	Target	Level
Understanding Earth and space	Knowledge and understanding	The Earth in space.	D
	Planning	Suggest possible outcomes to a planned investigation or experiment.	
	Collecting evidence	Observe events, noticing sequences and changes. Identify suitable sources to provide specific information for a given task.	D
	Recording and presenting	Record evidence in a variety of appropriate ways.	D
	Interpreting and evaluating	Draw conclusions and justify them with reference to evidence.	D

▲ Name _____

Solids, liquids and gases

A **solid** is something which usually does not change its shape, for example, a rock, sugar.
A **liquid** is something which can flow from one place to another, for example, water, milk.
A **gas** cannot usually be seen. It fills the whole space it is in, for example, the air around us.

▲ Look at the objects below. Decide whether each is a solid, liquid or gas.

▲ Make a list of the solids, liquids and gases in your classroom. Share your list with others. Do they agree?

butter	honey	wood	bubbles in soft drink
inside a balloon	salt	ice lolly	candle
ketchup	paper	steam	nail

▲ ESSENTIALS FOR SCIENCE: Changes

Changing solids, liquids and gases

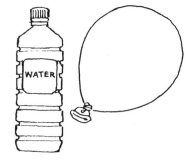

You will need: water; kettle; ice-tray; fruit juice; butter; saucepan; hotplate; baking powder; vinegar; sugar; jars; spoon; fridge; cup.

⚠ Adult supervision is needed for the heating experiments.

1 Boil some water. What happens?

2 Put some fruit juice in the freezer compartment of a fridge. Leave for several hours.

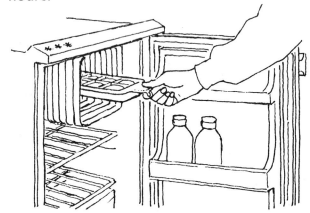

3 Put a teaspoon of baking powder into a jar. Add vinegar.

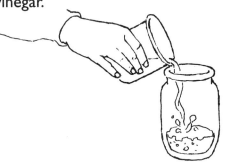

4 Heat some butter in a saucepan.

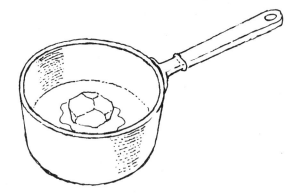

5 Boil some water. Add it to a cup with a teaspoon of sugar in it. Stir.

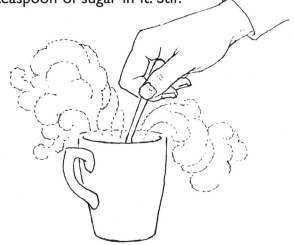

▲ Record your findings here.

Experiment	Substance	Action	Prediction – what will happen?	Result – what did it change to? solid? liquid? gas?
1	water	boil it		
2	fruit juice	freeze it		
3	baking powder	add vinegar		
4	butter	heat it		
5	sugar	add hot water		

Separating substances

You will need: salt; water; glass; spoon; saucepan; hotplate.

Some things are made from two or more substances. Sometimes it is necessary to separate them in order to obtain one of the substances. We can do this by evaporation and filtering.

▲ Try this for yourself.
⚠ Adult supervision is needed.

1 Mix several teaspoons of salt in a glass of water until the salt dissolves.

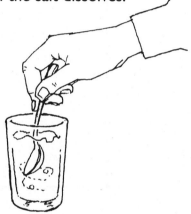

2 Pour the solution into a saucepan and boil the water.

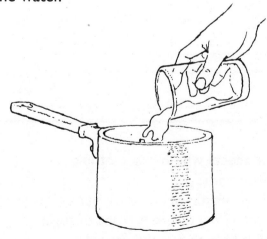

3 Observe what happens to the water. Where does it go? What is left over after the water has gone?

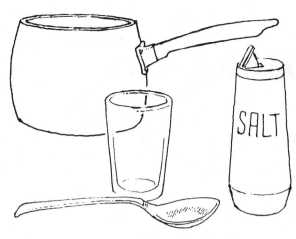

▲ Filtering
1 Set up a filter as in the diagram.
2 Fill the top with muddy water.
3 Watch the water which comes out. How has it changed?

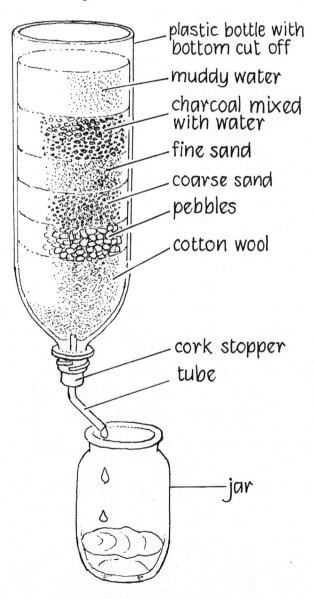

▲ Try out simpler filters such as paper, tights, socks, fabric. Which filter works best?

▲ Name _____

Dissolving things

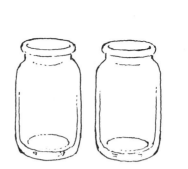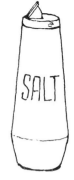

You will need: jam jars; water; sugar; salt; pepper; flour; scouring powder; bicarbonate of soda; spoon.

1 Fill a jar with water.
2 Add one spoonful of salt.
3 Stir.
4 Does the salt dissolve?

▲ Try out the other ingredients. Predict the result first then record what happens.

▲ Does the water change colour?

Substance	Prediction – will it dissolve?	Result
sugar		
salt		
pepper		
flour		
scouring powder		
bicarbonate of soda		

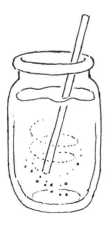

▲ What affects whether something dissolves or not?
▲ Do fine substances dissolve better than coarse ones? Try different types of sugar.
▲ Does it help to stir the water?
▲ Will heating the water affect how things dissolve?
▲ Which substance dissolves the fastest? Why do you think this is?

Physical and chemical changes

When we change the appearance of something without turning it into something else we are making a *physical change*, such as bending a nail or freezing water to make ice.

When we change something into something else we are making a *chemical change*, such as burning wood to make charcoal or smelting iron to make steel.

▲ Look at the following changes. Decide if there has been a physical or chemical change made. Discuss your decision with others. Do they agree?

▲ Make a list of physical and chemical changes which can be made at home or at school.

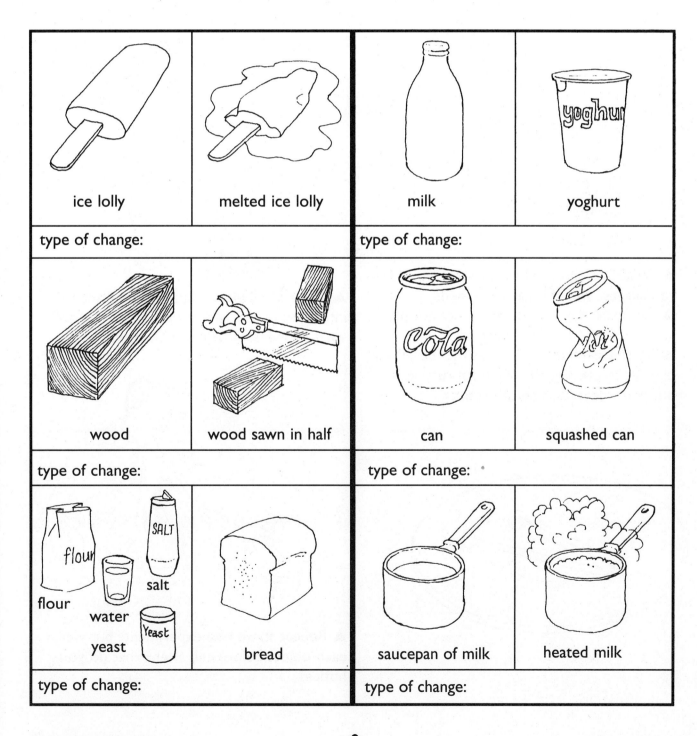

ice lolly	melted ice lolly	milk	yoghurt
type of change:		type of change:	
wood	wood sawn in half	can	squashed can
type of change:		type of change:	
flour, water, salt, yeast	bread	saucepan of milk	heated milk
type of change:		type of change:	

▲ ESSENTIALS FOR SCIENCE: Changes

▲ Name _____

Making chemical changes

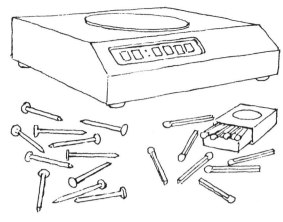

You will need: steel wool; saucer; water; nails; matches; saucer; paper; electronic scales.

Activity 1
▲ Soak some of the steel wool in water then place it on a saucer. Leave for several hours or overnight.

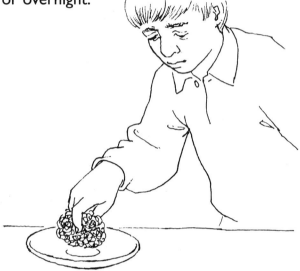

▲ What has happened to the steel wool? Can you suggest why this has happened?
▲ Compare this wool to the wool not placed in the water. Which is strongest?
▲ Try the same experiment with a nail. Think of ways to prevent the nail from rusting. Try out your ideas. Record the results.

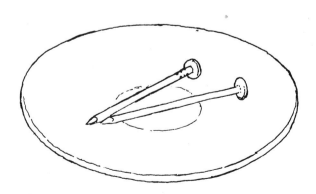

Activity 2
▲ Place a lighted match in a saucer and watch it burn. When cool, touch the match.
▲ What has happened to it? How has it changed?

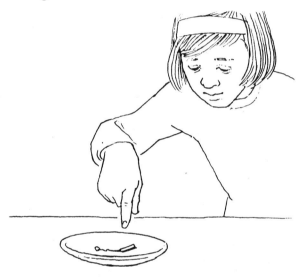

▲ Cut a small piece of paper and place this into the saucer. Light it with a match. Watch what happens. How has it changed?

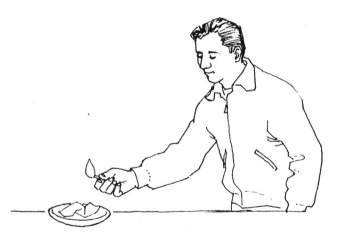

▲ Repeat these two experiments but weigh each object before and after. What do you notice?

Manufactured changes

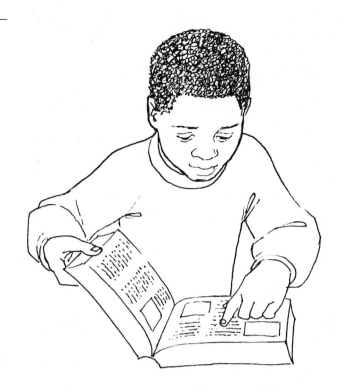

Humans are able to take a raw material found in nature, such as wood, and change it into something completely different. Wood can be manufactured into paper.

▲ Below is a group of things. For each object decide if it is a raw material or whether it has been changed (manufactured) in some way. Write your answer underneath each picture. You may need to discuss your ideas with a friend or use reference books to help you.

glass	diamond	oil	steel	iron ore
gold	plastic	wool	flour	aluminium
coal	salt	milk	petrol	silk

▲ ESSENTIALS FOR SCIENCE: Changes

▲ Name _____

Changing colours

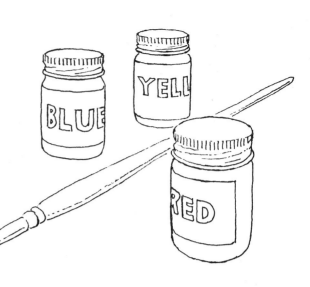

You will need: red, blue, yellow and white paint (or cellophane); paper; paint brush; card; felt-tipped pens; matchstick.

You can make different colours using two or three other colours mixed together.
▲ Try out these mixes:

Colour mix	Prediction – what colour will it make?	Result – what colour did it make?
blue and yellow		
red and yellow		
red and blue		
red, blue and yellow		
blue and white		
red and white		
yellow and white		

▲ How many different shades of each colour can you make?
▲ Can you make black?

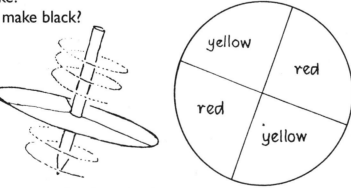

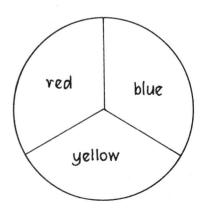

1 Now cut some circles from card.
2 Colour as shown with felt-tipped pens.
3 Make a hole in the centre for a matchstick.
4 Spin the cards quickly. What happens?

▲ Try different colours and patterns. Record the results.

▲ ESSENTIALS FOR SCIENCE: Changes

▲ Name _____

Chromatography

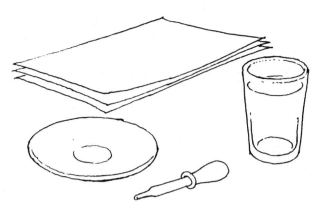

You will need: water-based felt-tipped pens; water; jars; blotting paper; food colouring; eye dropper; saucer.

Colours can be changed by mixing with other colours. Chromatography is a method used to separate all the colours which have been mixed together to make one colour.

Activity 1
1 Cut out a square of blotting paper (10cm x 10cm).
2 Draw a circle of any colour felt-tipped pen (or food colouring).
3 Place the paper over a saucer.
4 With an eye dropper, put one drop of water in the centre of the coloured dot.

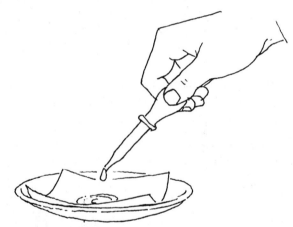

5 Wait until the ink stops spreading. Add another drop.
6 Repeat.
▲ What happens?

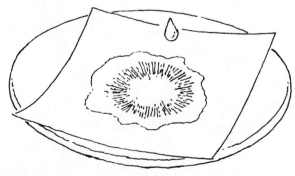

▲ Try out other colours and compare the results.

Activity 2
1 Cut out strips of blotting paper (33cm x 12 cm).
2 Place a dot of colour about 2cm from one end.

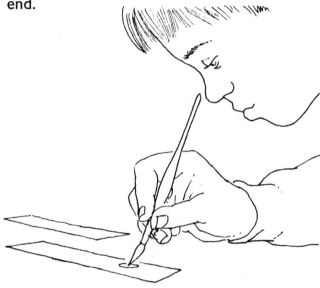

3 Put the strips into a jar of water so the dot of colour is just above the water line.
4 Watch what happens.
▲ Which colour uses the most mixtures?

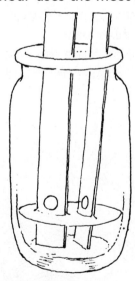

▲ Try out several different brands of the same colour, say, black. Do they all use the same colours to make black?

▲ ESSENTIALS FOR SCIENCE: Changes

▲ Name _____

Changing sounds

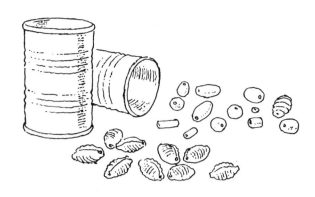

You will need: empty bottles; water; ice-cream cartons; rubber bands; tins; beads; pasta.

Sound is made when objects vibrate. We can change the pitch and loudness of the sound by altering the object making the sound. Pitch refers to how high or low the sound is.

▲ Find out more about pitch and loudness by making some musical instruments.
1 Fill bottles with different amounts of water.
2 Blow across the top of each bottle.
▲ How can you make the sounds higher/lower/louder?

5 Cut slits in the sides of an ice-cream carton at the top. Attach rubber bands and pluck these to make sounds.

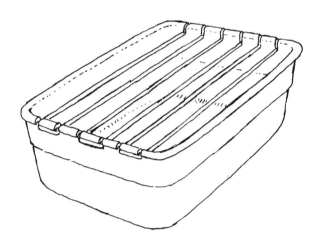

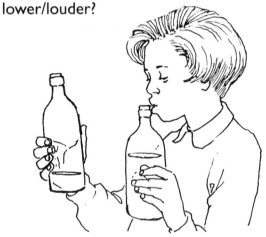

▲ How can you change the sounds? Try different sorts of rubber bands. Does it make a difference if the bands are raised by card?
▲ Can you make an instrument with bands of different lengths? How does this change the sounds made?

3 Fill tins with objects such as beads and pasta. Seal the end by placing card over it and secure with a rubber band.
4 Hit, shake, roll or rattle the tins.
▲ How can you change the sounds?

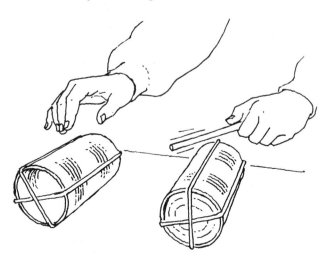

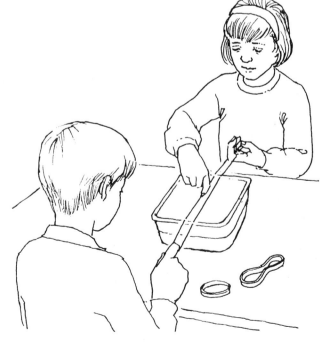

▲ ESSENTIALS FOR SCIENCE: Changes   14

▲ Name _____

Changes in strength

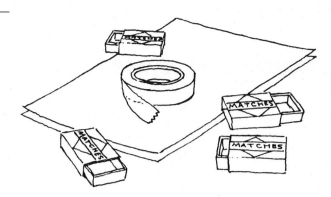

You will need: paper or thin card (A4 size); 4 matchboxes or blocks; measuring weights (1g – 1kg); sticky tape.

We can sometimes change the strength of something by altering its shape.

▲ Conduct this experiment to find out how the strength of paper can be changed.

▲ Use the paper in the following ways. See how much weight the paper will hold each time.

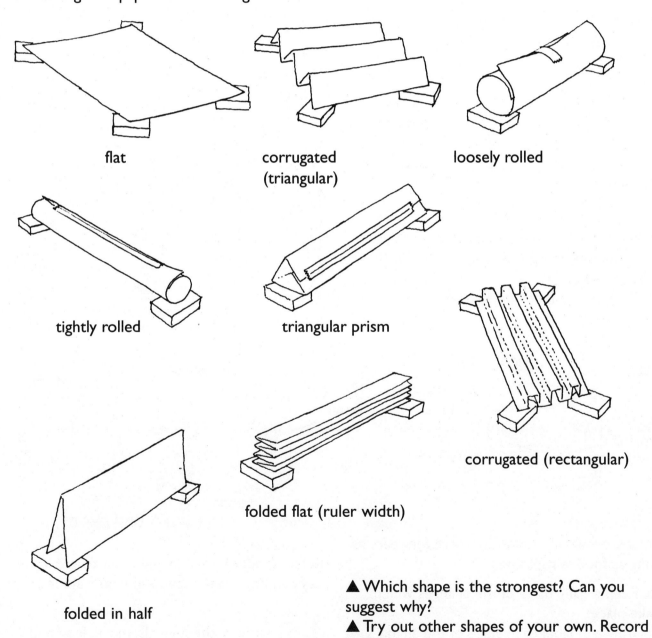

flat

corrugated (triangular)

loosely rolled

tightly rolled

triangular prism

corrugated (rectangular)

folded flat (ruler width)

folded in half

▲ Which shape is the strongest? Can you suggest why?
▲ Try out other shapes of your own. Record the results.
▲ How would these shapes affect how buildings or bridges are made?

▲ ESSENTIALS FOR SCIENCE: Changes

▲ Name _____

Animal life cycles

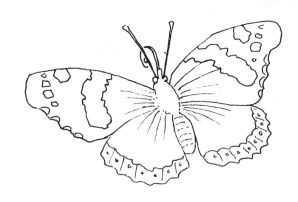

Some animals change completely as they grow. Many insects, such as butterflies and mealworms, do this. Frogs do too.

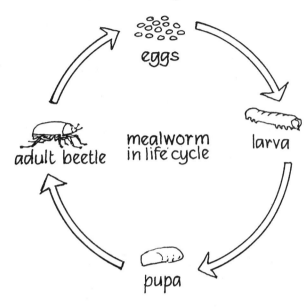

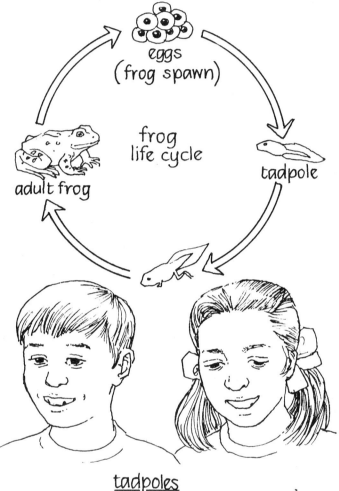

When animals change completely like this, it is called metamorphosis. You can watch these changes yourself.
▲ Prepare the following habitats:

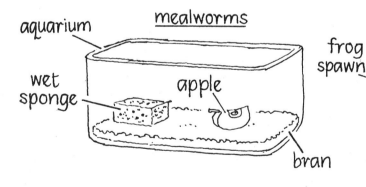

(Mealworms will happily live here for years as long as food is replaced.)

▲ Keep a daily diary of the changes which take place.
1 Draw and label each stage of the animal's life.
2 Write down questions you are keen to find out about.

(Release tadpoles when legs start to grow as they can no longer survive in water alone.)

3 Observe how the animals, move, feed and rest.
4 Do they prefer sunlight or shade?
5 Carefully measure the animals as they grow.

▲ ESSENTIALS FOR SCIENCE: Changes

How plants change

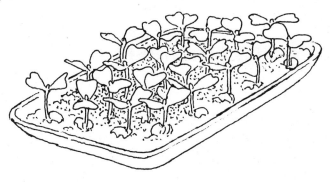

You will need: bean seeds; plant pot; soil.

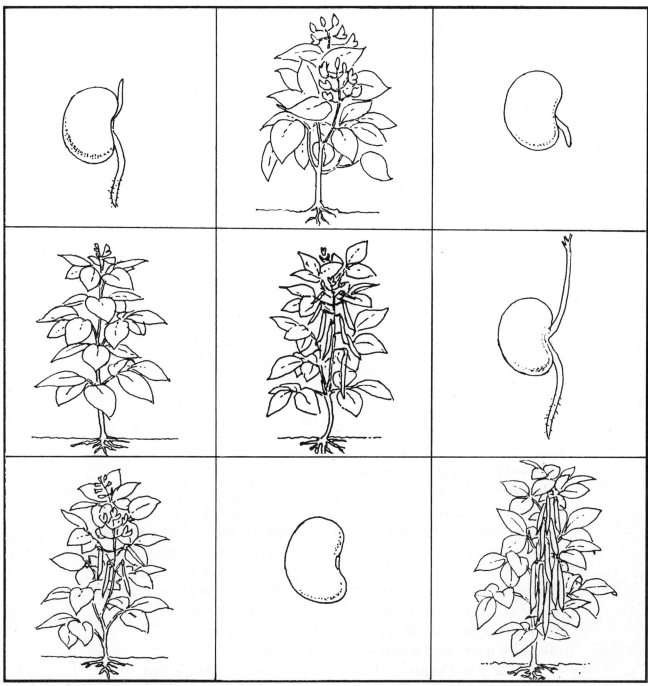

▲ How do plants change as they grow? Look at the pictures of a bean plant above. Cut out the pictures and place them in the correct order. Share you result with others. Do they agree?

▲ Plant some bean seeds in a plant pot in the classroom. Water when needed. Make a record of the plants' changes as they grow.

▲ Name _____

Photosynthesis

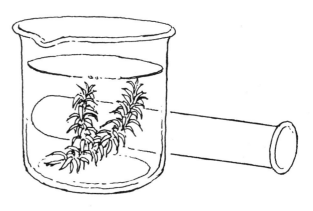

You will need: card; paper clips; water; methylated spirits; iodine; test-tube; funnel; beaker; pondweed.

Green plants are the only living things that can make their own food. They do this by using carbon dioxide from the air, water from the soil, energy from sunlight and a chemical called chlorophyll in the leaves. This process is called photosynthesis. The plant makes a type of sugar and it gives off oxygen into the air. The sugar helps the plant grow.

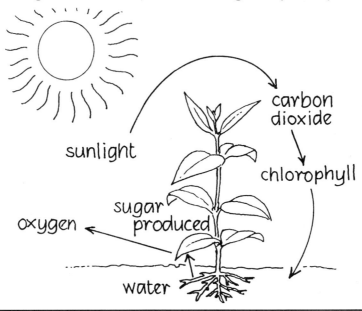

▲ Blocking sunlight – completely cover several leaves on a house-plant or tree – use card and attach with paper clips. After a week, examine the covered leaves. What do you notice? Why has this happened?

▲ Testing for sugar (starch) – cover only part of a leaf as above. Leave for several days (make sure it's sunny). Boil the leaf for a few seconds, then place the leaf in a solution of 70% methylated spirits and 30% water (an adult should do this). Now cover the leaf with iodine. (Adult supervision is needed.) What do you notice?

▲ To show oxygen is produced – place some Canadian pondweed in an upturned funnel in a beaker of pond water (as shown). Place a test-tube over the end of the funnel. Place it in sunlight. What happens? Place it in the dark. What happens?

▲ Set up your own experiments to show that plants need water and sunlight to grow. Record your results.

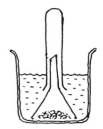

▲ ESSENTIALS FOR SCIENCE: Changes

▲ Name _____

Will it rot?

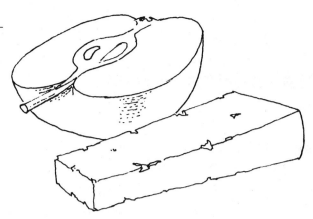

You will need: plastic food bags with ties; cheddar cheese; apples; cotton wool; water; hand lenses.

▲ Find out what happens to food kept in different conditions by doing this experiment.

1 Place a piece of cheese into three different bags.
2 Seal.
3 Place one bag in the fridge (a), one in a warm spot (b) (near a heater, sunny window ledge) and one in the room away from the sun (c).

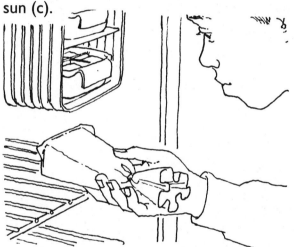

4 Do the same with pieces of apple.
5 Soak some cotton wool in water then place this in a bag with some cheese.
6 Seal.
7 In another bag, place some cheese which has been rubbed on the floor.

8 Seal.
9 Place both bags in position C.
10 Do the same with the apple.
11 Predict what might happen in each case.
▲ Record the results. Make daily observations. Note changes in colour, shape and texture.

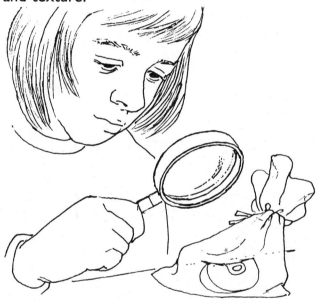

▲ Does anything grow on the food? What is it?

Note: When observing, do not open the bags. Use a hand lens to look closely through the plastic bag.

▲ Write down the things which you think help food to rot. How can it be prevented?

▲ ESSENTIALS FOR SCIENCE: Changes

▲ Name _____

Making compost

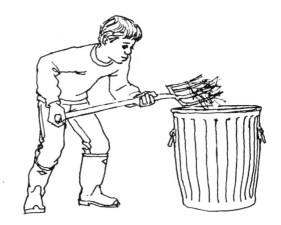

You will need: plastic rubbish bin with a lid; soil; grass clippings; leaves (not evergreen); vegetable and fruit waste; garden fork.

We can change food waste, which we would normally throw away, into something useful: we can make it into compost.

▲ Try making compost yourself.
1 Make holes in the bin and lid.
2 Layer the bin as follows: grass clippings and soil, vegetable/fruit waste, rotting leaves, soil... repeating until the bin is full.

3 Put on the lid and keep the bin in a sunny spot where air can get in from the sides.
4 Mix the layers regularly with a garden fork.
▲ Observe the compost every few days. Record what happens.

▲ Try out the compost when it is ready (it will be dark and crumbly). Plant two bean seeds. Use compost on one and garden soil or sand with the other. Record the results. Which bean grows best?

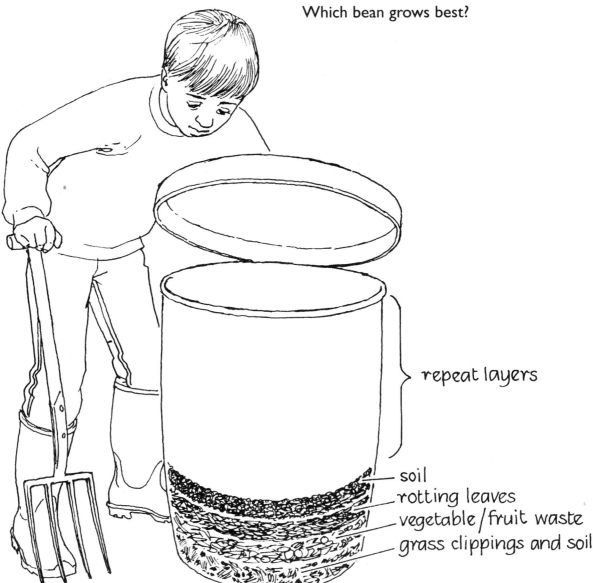

▲ ESSENTIALS FOR SCIENCE: Changes

▲ Name _____

Genetics

Genetics is the science which studies the traits of animals and plants which are passed on to the next generation. In your own family, for example, all family members might have fair hair. As the family members grow and have their own families some of these traits may change.

▲ Find out what common traits your family has and what has been changed over the years.

▲ Try and complete as much of the table as you can. Rely on photographs and people's memories if necessary!

Family member	Colour of eyes	Colour of hair	Freckles?	Free ear-lobes?	Turned up nose?
Me					
My father					
My brother or sister					
My father's father					
My father's mother					
My father's sister or brother					
My mother					
My mother's father					
My mother's mother					
My mother's sister or brother					
My cousin					
My nephew or niece					

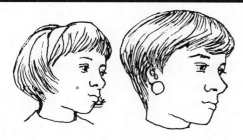

▲ Who are you most like? Does your family have a common trait or have there been changes in the way your family looks?

▲ ESSENTIALS FOR SCIENCE: Changes

Fossils

You will need: plaster of Paris; water; Vaseline; shell; small carton such as a milk container; modelling clay; leaves.

Fossils are traces of animals or plants found in rocks. The animals and plants lived on Earth millions of years ago. Scientists use fossils to learn how living things have changed over time. They can also show how land forms have changed, for example sometimes fossils of shells are found in deserts, which tell us that the desert area was once under water.

Activity 1
Make your own fossil.
1 Mix the plaster with water until it is quite thick.
2 Pour the mixture into the carton until it is 2/3 full.
3 Coat the shell with Vaseline.
4 When the plaster begins to harden place the shell into the plaster.
5 Let it set.
6 Remove the shell.
7 Rub Vaseline over the shell dent and the top of the hard plaster.
8 Mix some more plaster of Paris and pour it into the carton.
9 When dry, lift off the top layer carefully. You have a 'fossil' cast.

Activity 2
1 Make the clay into a slab about 1cm thick.
2 Carefully press a leaf into the clay.
3 Remove.
4 Allow the clay to harden.

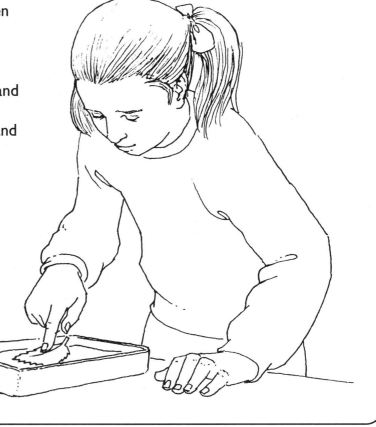

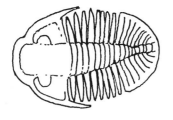

▲ Find out how real fossils are formed.

Changes in the landscape – 1

Erosion is the name given to the process where land is worn away. Erosion is caused by water, wind and ice. Over time, the landscape can change greatly due to this wearing away.

▲ Look at the diagrams below. Decide how the land has been worn away. Look at the landscape features produced. Decide how they may have been formed. Use reference books to help you.

Landscape features		Your comments
1. before / after		Type of erosion _____
2. before / after		Type of erosion _____
3. before / after		Type of erosion _____

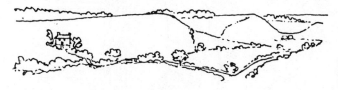

▲ Look at landscape features in your area. Decide how they were formed.

ESSENTIALS FOR SCIENCE: Changes

▲ Name _____

Weathering

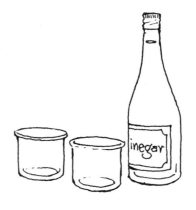

You will need: chalk (not blackboard chalk); vinegar; water; 2 small containers.

The surfaces of rocks and buildings can be changed by weathering. Weathering is a wearing away of the surface. It is usually caused by wind and rain but can also be caused by pollution in the air (acid rain) and the freezing and thawing of ice in rock cracks.

▲ Investigate the effects of acid rain yourself.

1 Place two pieces of chalk the same length into a container each.
2 Cover one piece of chalk with water and one piece with vinegar.

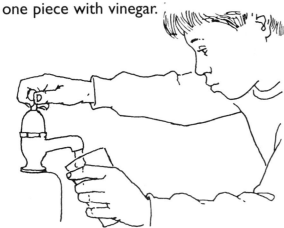

3 Watch closely. What do you notice?
4 Leave the containers overnight.
5 Empty the containers and observe any differences in the pieces of chalk.
▲ Is one piece easier to break?
▲ Is one piece smaller or softer?

6 Can you explain what has happened?

_____
_____
_____
_____
_____
_____
_____

▲ Take a walk around your neighbourhood and note or photograph any evidence of weathering on buildings in your area.

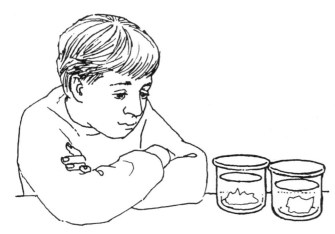
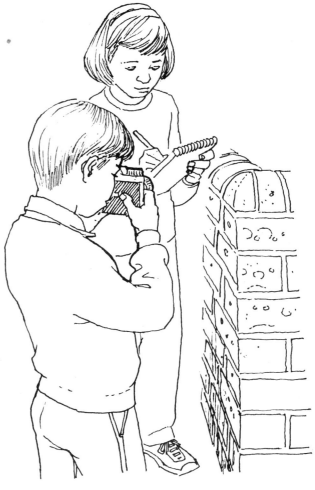

▲ ESSENTIALS FOR SCIENCE: Changes

▲ Name _____

Changes in the landscape – 2

Humans are able to carry out activities which can dramatically change the landscape. Sometimes these changes improve the environment for the plants and animals which live there and sometimes the changes can destroy important habitats.

▲ Look at the diagrams below. Decide whether an improvement or a destruction of the landscape has taken place. Consider also how the activities have affected the plants and animals living there.

Human activity		Your comments
1. before	after	
2. before	after	
3. before	after	

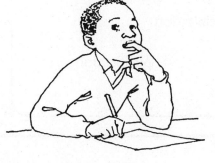

▲ Make a list of human activities which have improved or destroyed habitats for plants and animals where you live.

▲ ESSENTIALS FOR SCIENCE: Changes

▲ Name _____

The water cycle

Water is continually moving into the atmosphere by evaporation. It returns to earth in the form of snow, rain, dew and hail. On the way, water is used and changed in some way by plants and animals, including humans.

▲ Using reference books to help you, decide which word from the box describes each stage in the water cycle diagram. Some words may be used more than once.

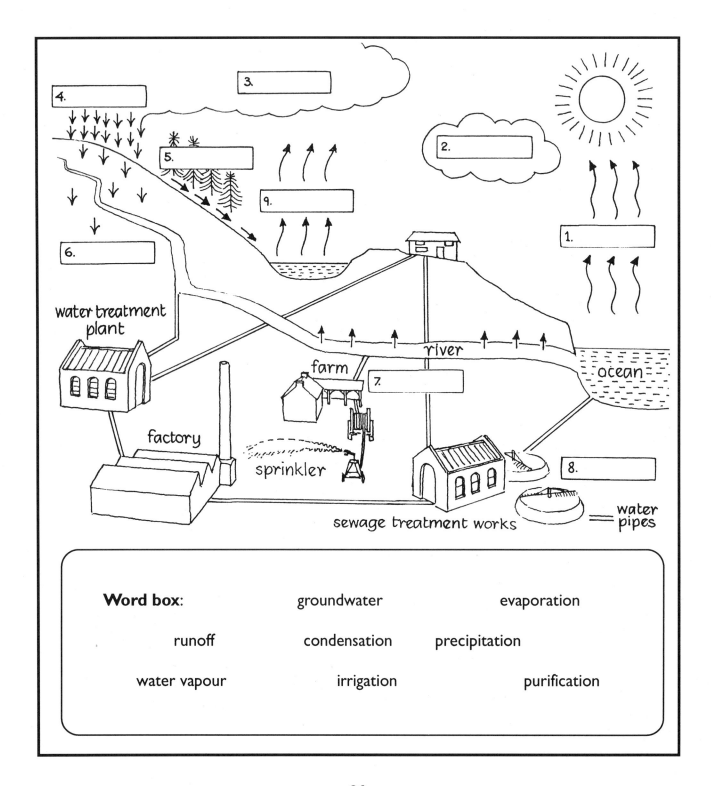

Word box: groundwater   evaporation   runoff   condensation   precipitation   water vapour   irrigation   purification

▲ ESSENTIALS FOR SCIENCE: Changes

Changes in the weather – temperature

You will need: an alcohol thermometer.

Temperature is a measure of how hot or cold something is. It is measured in degrees Celsius (°C) or degrees Fahrenheit (°F). A thermometer containing mercury or alcohol is used to measure temperature. As temperature increases, the mercury or alcohol expands in the glass tube and its level rises.

▲ Air temperature is always measured in the shade – the following experiment will help you find out why.
1 Measure the temperature in the shade and in direct sunlight at different times of the day.
2 Record your results in the chart.

▲ Which temperatures are higher? in shade? or in sun? Why do you think this is?
▲ What time of day is the hottest?
▲ Is it always hottest at this time each day?
▲ What is the average temperature for the day? for the week?

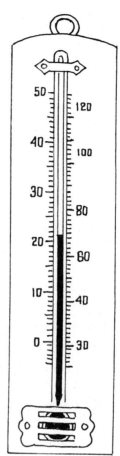

▲ If possible, record over several weeks to find the average temperature for the month.

Condition and time	Monday	Tuesday	Wednesday	Thursday	Friday
9.00am – shade					
9.00am – in sun					
10.30am – shade					
10.30am – in sun					
12.00pm – shade					
12.00pm – in sun					
3.00pm – in shade					
3.00pm – in sun					

▲ Name _____

Changes in the weather – wind speed and rainfall

You will need: plastic funnel; plastic bottle; Plasticine; tray of sand; measuring jar.

A simple way to determine wind speed is to use the Beaufort wind scale.
An approximate speed can be calculated by observing the effect wind has on things around us. See the table below.

▲ Make a rain gauge.
1 Stand the plastic bottle in the tray of sand.
2 Put the funnel in the neck of the bottle.
3 Fix it in place with the Plasticine.
4 Place outside to catch the rain.
5 Empty the collected rain daily into the measuring jar.
6 Record the results on the table.

▲ Record daily wind speed and rainfall.
▲ Work out the average weekly rainfall.

Day	Amount of rainfall	Wind speed (Beaufort force)
1		
2		
3		
4		
5		
6		
7		
8		
9		
10		
11		
12		
13		
14		

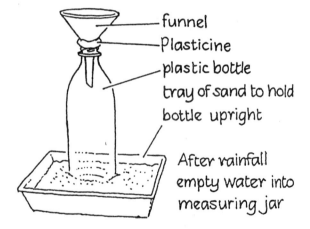

funnel
Plasticine
plastic bottle
tray of sand to hold bottle upright
After rainfall empty water into measuring jar

Beaufort wind scale		
Beaufort Force	Wind speed (in km/h) 10 m above ground	Description
0	Less than 1	Calm: Smoke rises vertically
1	1-5	Light Air: Not enough to move wind vane, but smoke drifts with the wind
2	6-11	Light Breeze: Wind felt on face, leaves rustle, and wind vane moves
3	12-19	Gentle Breeze: Leaves and small twigs move and light flags extended
4	20-28	Moderate Breeze: Raises dust and loose paper. Small branches move
5	29-39	Fresh Breeze: Small trees in leaf sway
6	40-50	Strong Breeze: Large branches move. Difficult to use umbrella
7	51-61	Near Gale: Whole trees sways. Uncomfortable to walk against the wind
8	62-74	Gale: Twigs break off trees. Difficult to walk against the wind
9	75-88	Strong Gale: Slight damage to buildings. May blow shingles off roof
10	89-102	Storm: Tree uprooted. Considerable damage
11	103-117	Violent Storm: Widespread damage
12	118 and over	Hurricane: Very rare inland. Violent destruction

▲ Name _____

Changes in the weather – wind direction

You will need: piece of thick card cut into the shape of an arrow; a long pin; small bead; pencil with eraser; compass.

Wind vanes are used to determine wind direction. Wind carries with it changes in the weather. Winds are named after the direction from which they blow – a wind blowing from the north towards the south is called northerly wind.

A wind rose (as shown below) can be used to show the direction from which the wind most often comes. This is called a prevailing wind.

▲ Make a wind vane (as shown on the right) to find out wind direction.
1 At the same time each day, take your wind vane outside to find out the wind direction.
2 Colour in a square on the wind rose each day for the wind's direction.
3 At the end of the week, the direction with the most squares coloured in will show the prevailing wind direction.

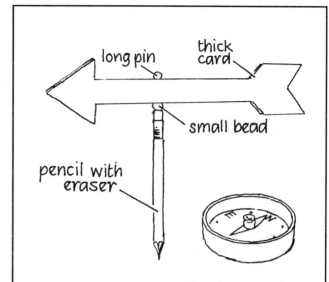

1 Fix the arrow of card to the pencil as shown in the diagram.
2 The arrow will point towards the direction the wind is blowing from.
3 Use a compass to find out the direction.

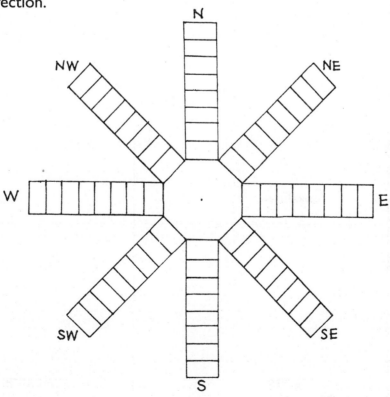

▲ ESSENTIALS FOR SCIENCE: Changes

▲ Name _____

The seasons

The changing seasons have an effect on the plants and animals around us.
▲ Find out about the animals and plants below.

▲ Draw or write what they look like/what happens to them each season.
▲ How do the seasons affect you? Write down how you feel, what you wear, what you do for each season.

Autumn	hedgehog	beech
Winter	holly	stoat
Spring	swallow	daffodil
Summer	grass	Atlantic salmon

▲ ESSENTIALS FOR SCIENCE: Changes

Day and night

What changes take place with plants, animals and humans during the day and night?

▲ Look at the pictures below. List all the changes which might occur if it was night time.

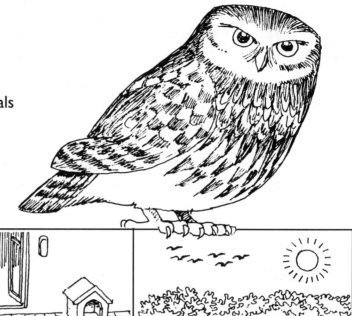

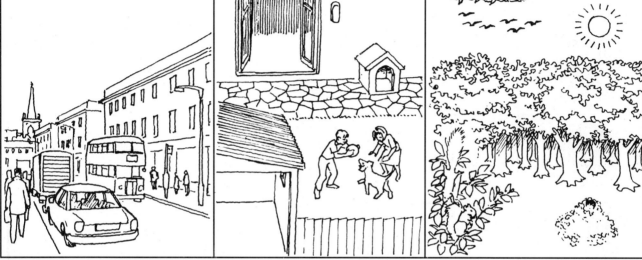

▲ Now list all the changes which might occur in these pictures if it was daytime.

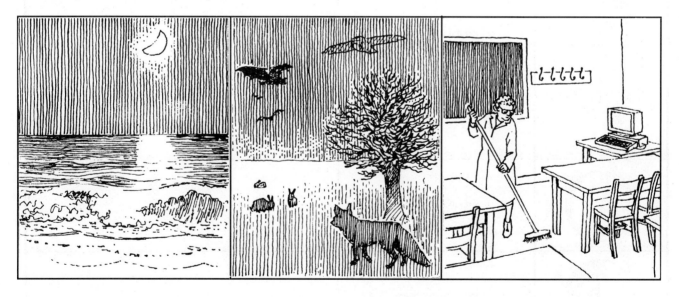

▲ Record the sunrise and sunset times for one month (use newspapers or contact the meteorological station near you)
▲ Calculate the numbers of hours of daylight each day.

▲ What do you notice about the number of hours as the month progresses? Can you suggest why?
▲ Find out what causes day and night.

▲ ESSENTIALS FOR SCIENCE: Changes

▲ Name _____

Changes in the moon

Throughout each month the moon appears to change shape. Can you suggest why?

▲ Look at each moon shape. Draw a diagram to show how this shape has been caused. The first one has been done for you.

▲ Try to watch the moon changes at night from where you live. Record the changing shapes.

Moon phase	Name of phase	Why it looks like this
	new	sun ○ E
	crescent	
	first quarter (half)	
	gibbous	
	full	
	gibbous	
	last quarter	
	crescent	

▲ ESSENTIALS FOR SCIENCE: Changes